Diabetic Diet: A Complete Step

By Step Guide for Beginners

Contents

Diabetes Diet & Food Tips

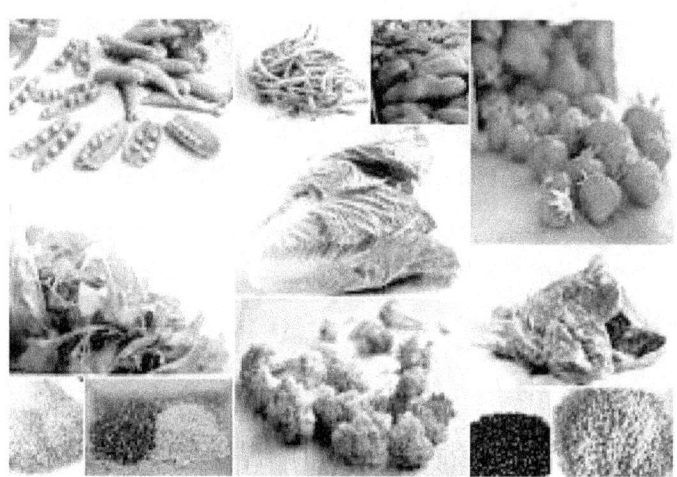

Diabetes cases are on the rise but most cases are preventable with healthy lifestyle changes. While eating right is important, one can still enjoy one's favorite foods and take pleasure from meals without feeling hungry or deprived.

Small changes equal big results

Whether you're trying to prevent or control diabetes, you can make a big difference with healthy lifestyle changes. The most important thing for your health is to lose weight; losing about 5% to 10% of your total weight can help you lower your blood sugar, your blood pressure and cholesterol levels. It's easy to make positive changes even after you've already developed diabetes.

What you need to know about diabetes and your diet

A diabetes diet is a healthy eating plan that is high in nutrients, low in fat, and moderate in calories; it is a healthy diet for everyone. For this reason, one needs to pay more attention to the food choices one makes.

Diabetes and diet tip 1: Choose high-fiber, slow-release Carbs

Carbohydrates have a big impact on blood sugar levels when compared to fats and protein. One must limit highly refined carbohydrates like white bread, pasta, rice and snack foods. Carbohydrates are the best choice for the diabetes diet as they keep blood sugar levels even as these are digested more slowly and can prevent the body from producing too much insulin.

Make the Glycemic index easy

The glycemic index (GI) tells how quickly a food can turn into sugar when it enters your body. High GI foods increase the blood sugar in your body faster than the low GI foods that have less of an effect. The foods can be classified into three broad categories: fire, water, and coal. The foods that are harder to break by the body are considered to be best for your health.

Fire foods include white foods (white rice, white pasta, white bread, potatoes, and most baked goods), sweets, chips, etc. They have a high GI and are low in fiber and protein. They should be included in your diet in limited amounts.

Water foods can be eaten as many times as you like. They include all vegetables and most types of fruit but not canned ones.

Coal foods like nuts, lean meats, whole grains, and beans can especially include whole-wheat products that have a low GI and are high in protein.

Diabetes and diet tip 2: Be smart about sweets

Eating for diabetes doesn't mean eliminating sugar. If you have diabetes, you can still enjoy a small serving of your favorite dessert now and then but with moderation. Once your eating habits become healthier that foods which you used to love may seem too rich or too sweet, you may start looking yourself for healthier options in your diet.

How to include sweets in a diabetes-friendly diet

Cut down on eating bread (or rice or pasta) if you want dessert. Eating sweets at a meal adds extra carbohydrates to your diet. Thus, it is best to cut back on the other carb-containing foods in the same meal.

Add some healthy fat to your dessert. Fat slows down the digestive process and the blood sugar levels don't spike as quickly. You can include healthy fats like yogurt into your diet.

Eat sweets with a meal and not as a stand-alone snack. When eaten alone, sweets and desserts can cause your blood sugar levels to rise. But if eaten along with other healthy foods, your blood sugar will be in control.

When you eat dessert, truly savor each bite. When you indulgence in your favorite dessert, eat slowly and pay attention to the flavors and textures because you'll enjoy it more and will not overeat.

Tricks for cutting down on sugar

Reduce the number of soft drinks, sodas and juice you drink. According to a recent study, beverage servings increase the risk of diabetes as they contain artificial sweeteners; this is not good for the health. Reduce the intake of creamers and sweeteners in tea and coffee drinks. Reduce foods that involve sweeteners like iced tea, yogurt, and oatmeal.

Find healthy ways to satisfy your sweet tooth. Try to reduce your craving for sweets. Instead, find some healthy ways. Natural sugars in fruits still are less likely to cause any harm.

Diabetes and your diet tip 3: Choose fats wisely

Fats in a limited quantity are necessary for the body. People with diabetes are at a higher risk for heart disease so it is essential that you monitor fats in your diet. Some fats are unhealthy whereas others have huge health benefits. Since all fats are high in calories, one should always watch for the intake amount.

Unhealthy fats – Trans fats and saturated fats are unhealthy fats. Animal products such as red meat, whole milk dairy products, and eggs constitute the saturated fats. Trans fats are mostly used by manufacturers of food products that prevent the food from getting spoiled and are bad for your health.

Healthy fats – The best fats are unsaturated fats that include olive oil, canola oil, nuts, and avocados among other stuff which come from plant and fish sources and are liquid at room temperature.

Diabetes and diet tip 4: Eat regularly and keep a food diary

To avoid diabetes, develop a habit of eating regularly and maintain a diary that will help you to analyze what you eat and how healthy it is. Not just that, you will also be able to keep your weight in check.

Maintain a regular meal schedule:

By maintaining a regular meal schedule, your body can regulate blood sugar levels and weight in a better manner. Don't skip breakfast; have a good and healthy breakfast. Eat breakfast every day; it will help you gain energy. Eat regular small meals—up to 6 per day. People tend to overeat when they are very hungry, so eating at regular intervals will help you to keep your blood glucose levels in control. Keep calorie intakes the same. Eat the same amount of calories every day, avoid overeating at one meal.

Diabetic diet

A diabetic diet is recommended in order to control blood sugar levels. The diet should be high in dietary fiber, low in fat and low in sugar. Diabetics are encouraged to reduce their carbohydrate intake.

However, some dietitians today recommend a typical healthy diet: one high in fiber, with a variety of fruit and vegetables, and low in both sugar and fat, especially saturated fat.

Carbohydrates

Dieticians recommend that carbohydrates for diabetics should be complex carbohydrates.

Low-carbohydrate alternatives

Some studies show that a low-carbohydrate diet can be effective in the dietary management of type 2 diabetes and can also prevent blood sugar levels from rising.

Vegan/vegetarian

The incidence of diabetes is lower in vegetarians. These studies have shown that a vegan diet is effective in managing type2 diabetes. It is beneficial for diabetics to go vegetarian as this can help you to cut down on saturated fats. It is recommended for diabetics to have eight portions of fruit and vegetable a day. They have high levels of dietary fiber.

Timing of meals

For diabetics, healthy eating is not simply a matter of "what one eats", but also *when* one eats. It is necessary to eat at regular intervals in order to keep your blood sugar levels in check.

Alcohol and drugs

Alcohol must be consumed in moderation. Diabetics should not consume alcohol on an empty stomach and should take some starchy food such as potato crisps with the consumption of alcohol.

Specific diets

The *Pritikin Diet* consists of fruit, vegetables, whole grains high in carbohydrates and roughage. The diet should be accompanied by exercise which is vital for any diabetic patient to reduce sugar levels.

G.I. Diet – A low glycemic index of one's diet helps to improve and control diabetes. Use multi-grain and breads, legumes and whole grains—foods that convert slowly to glucose.

Low Carb Diet – Carbohydrates must be replaced with fatty foods such as nuts, seeds, meats, fish, oils, eggs, avocados, olives, and vegetables that will help to reverse diabetes.

High fiber diet – A high fiber diet works better and controls blood sugar levels.

Paleolithic diet – The Paleolithic diet improves glucose tolerance in humans with type 2 diabetes.

Vegan diet – A low-fat vegan diet improves glycemic control.

Diabetes diet- Create your healthy-eating plan

An diabetes diet is a healthy-eating plan that helps to control blood sugar.

A diabetes diet is medically known as medical nutrition therapy (MNT) for diabetes which translates into eating nutritious foods in moderation and at regular intervals.

A diabetes diet or MNT is a healthy eating plan rich in nutrients and low in fat and calories, where fruits, vegetables and whole grains should form an important part of the diet.

Purpose

MNT helps you to control your blood sugar level and weight control if you are diabetic. Excess calories and fat can create an undesirable rise in blood glucose.

Make healthy food choices and track your eating habits as this will help to manage your blood glucose level and keep it within a safe range. For people with type 2 diabetes, weight loss makes it easier to control blood glucose and offers a host of other health benefits.

Recommended foods

Take nutritious foods to control your sugar levels.

Healthy carbohydrates- During digestion, sugar and starches break down into blood glucose. Take carbohydrates such as fruits, vegetables, whole grains, legumes (beans, peas and lentils) and low-fat dairy products.

Fiber-rich foods- Dietary fiber is included in all parts of the plant and can decrease the risk of heart disease and help control blood sugar levels.

'Good' fats- Foods that have monounsaturated as well as polyunsaturated fats can keep your cholesterol levels in check.

Foods to avoid

There are many foods to watch for including:

Saturated fats- High-fat products like hot dogs and bacon contain saturated fats. Only 7% should make for the total calories you consume.

Trans fats- These are found in processed snacks and baked goods and should be avoided completely.

Cholesterol- High-fat dairy products and high-fat animal proteins, egg yolks, shellfish, liver, and other organ meats are sources for cholesterol. 300 milligrams (mg) of cholesterol a day is enough.

Sodium - Aim for less than 2,300 mg of sodium a day.

Putting it all together: Creating a plan

Counting carbohydrates- Carbohydrates break down into glucose and affect the blood glucose level. Make sure your intake amount of carbohydrates is the same each day when you take diabetes medications. Your blood glucose level is likely to fluctuate more otherwise.

The exchange system- Using the exchange system is recommended as it groups foods into categories like carbohydrates, meats and fats. For instance, for one carbohydrate serving you can exchange a small apple for a 1/3 cup of cooked pasta. An exchange has same amount of carbohydrates, fats, proteins and calories.

Glycemic index- Foods that have high glycemic index numbers are associated with greater increases in blood sugar than foods with low glycemic index numbers.

If you are diabetic, your body is not able to properly use insulin which leads to high blood glucose or blood sugar levels. Healthy eating keeps blood sugar levels in a good target range. It is an essential part to manage your diabetes as controlling blood sugar can prevent the complications of diabetes from being worse.

A registered dietitian can help to make an effective eating plan for you taking into account your weight, medicines, lifestyle, and other health problems.

Healthy diabetic eating plans can include these important strategies:

a. Limit foods that are high in sugar

b. Eat smaller quantities in the day

c. Be careful about how many carbohydrates you eat

d. Eat a variety of whole-grain foods, fruits and vegetables daily

e. Eat less fat

f. Limit your use of alcohol

g. Use less salt

Eating Considerations

You'll have an easier time with staying healthy if you think about the following:

a. What your body needs

b. How much you need

c. When to have it

You must especially make the right food selection so that you can:

a. Feel good every day

b. Lose weight

c. Lower your risk for heart disease, stroke, and other problems caused by diabetes

d. Keep your blood glucose in your control.

e. Keep from being reliant on diabetes medicines help.

Next, you will see that you can prevent health problems by keeping your blood glucose levels in control.

Blood Glucose Levels

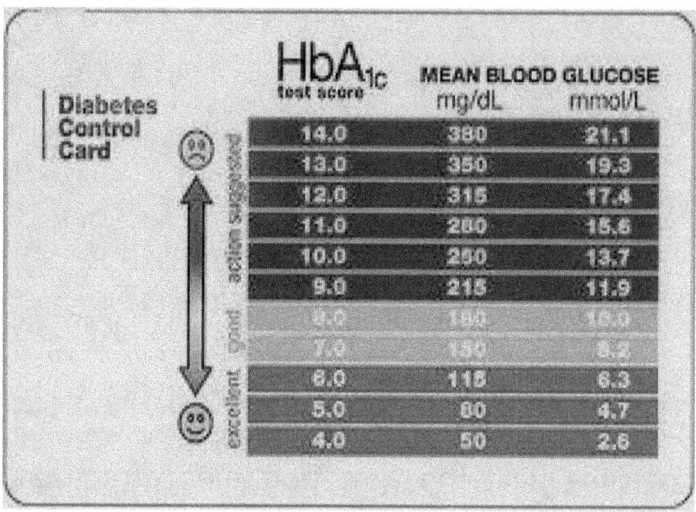

What should my blood glucose levels be?

These are the target blood glucose levels for people with Diabetes:

- Before meals -70 to 130

- 1 to 2 hours -less than 180

- After the start of a meal

How can I keep my blood glucose levels on target?

You can keep your blood glucose levels on target by:

- Using wise food choices

- Being physically active

- Taking medicines on time

- Following a schedule for meals

- Developing a physical activity plan with plenty of regular exercise

Keep the following points in mind:

a. Ask your doctor what kind of exercises can be suitable for you.

b. After exercising, check your feet for redness or sores. Consult your doctor if your sores do not heal. Warm up for 5 to 10 minutes before you begin exercise. Begin with walking slowly first, stretch, and then walk faster. Walk slowly again to finish your exercise.

c. If your blood glucose level is high, Ask your doctor whether you should exercise or not.

d. Know the signs of low blood glucose and observe them as they appear.

e. Find an exercise buddy. Many people find they are more likely to do something active if a friend joins them.

Low Blood Glucose (Hypoglycemia)

Low blood sugar levels can you feel weak, confused, irritable or tired and get a headache and sweat. Check your blood glucose, if you feel these symptoms are occurring with yourself.

If your blood glucose level is below 70, just have one of the following to correct it:

a. 3 or 4 glucose tablets

b. 1/2 cup (4 ounces) of any fruit juice

c. 1/2 cup (4 ounces) of a regular soft drink

d. 1 cup (8 ounces) of milk

The Diabetes Food Pyramid

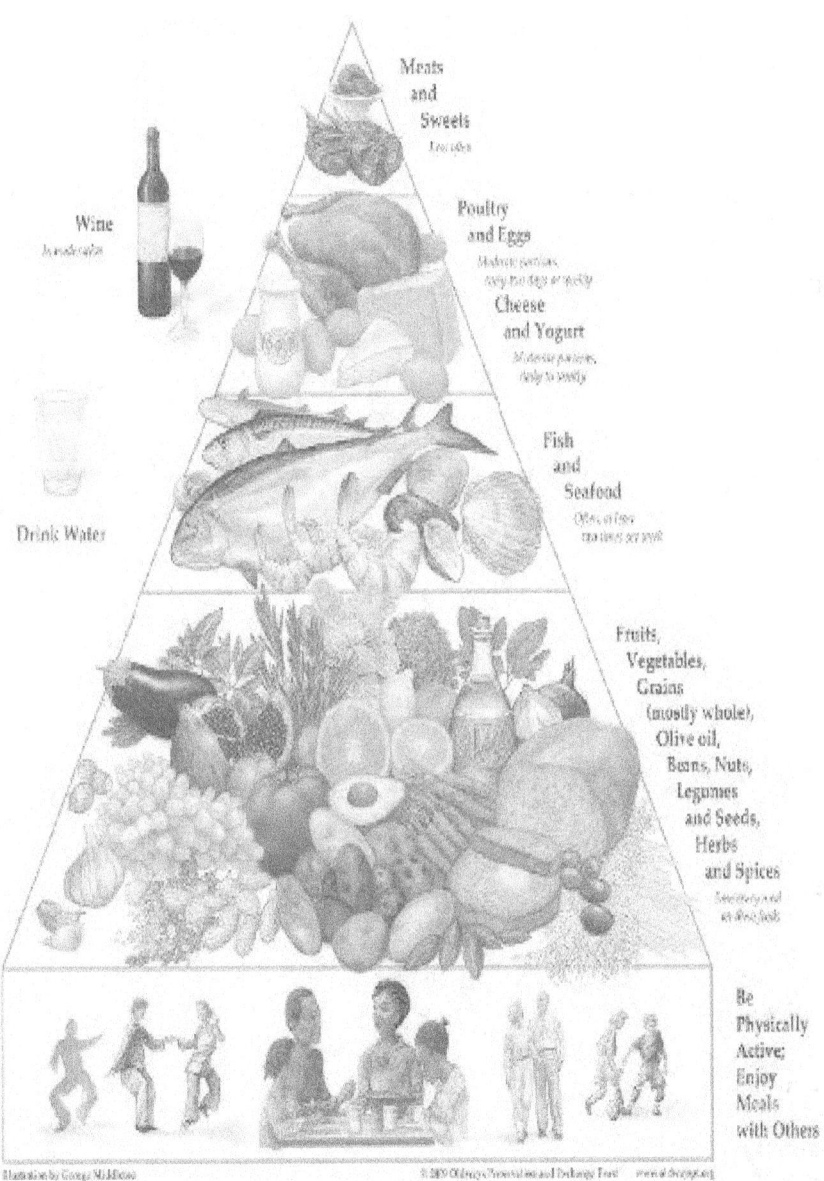

The diabetes food pyramid is one that helps you to make wise food

choices. It divides foods into groups on the basis of what it contains.

Foods that contain the starches, fruits, vegetables, and milk groups are highest in carbohydrates which affect the blood glucose levels the most.

How much should I eat each day?

a. Eat about 1,200 to 1,600 calories in a day for the best results. This is especially the case if you are a small woman who needs exercise or a medium-sized woman who might be more likely to gain weight over time.

You need 1,200 to 1,600 calories from these categories in your daily routine:

- 6 starches, 2 milks
- 3 vegetables, 4 to 6 ounces meat

Make Your Own Diabetes Food Pyramid

Include the following in your food pyramid:

Starches

Starches are included in bread, grains, cereal, pasta, and vegetables like corn and potatoes. Along with starches, they also provide carbohydrates, vitamins, minerals, and fiber. Whole grain starches have more vitamins, minerals, and fiber, thereby making it healthier. Eating food that contains starches is healthy for diabetics and everyone.

Some starches to be aware of include the following:

- Bread

- Pasta

- Corn

- Potatoes

- Rice

- Crackers

- Cereal

- Beans

How much starch goes into one serving?

1 small potato + 1 small corn or 2 slices of bread

1 small roll +1/2 cup of peas+ 1 small potato or 1 cup of rice

How can you eat starches the right way?

a. Eat whole grain products.

b. Eat less, French fries, pastries, or biscuits among other unhealthy

   starches.

c. Use low-fat yogurt or fat-free cream.

d. Use mustard and not mayonnaise in a sandwich.

e. Use low-fat or fat-free substitutes mayonnaise.

f. Eat cereal with fat-free (skim) milk.

Vegetables

Vegetables are rich in vitamins, minerals, and fiber and are low in carbohydrates. Examples of vegetables to use include the following:

- Lettuce

- Broccoli

- Spinach

- Peppers

- Carrots

- Green beans

- Tomatoes

- Celery

What does a serving consist of?

½ cup cooked carrots or ½ cup cooked green beans or 1 cup salad

½ cup cooked carrots + 1 cup salad or ½ cup vegetable juice + ½ cup cooked green beans

½ cup cooked green beans + ½ cup cooked green beans and 1 small tomato or ½ cup broccoli + 1 cup tomato sauce

What are the best ways for you to eat vegetables?

a. Eat fat-free vegetables that are cooked properly. Raw vegetables especially work the best.

b. Try low-fat salad dressing if you are to use it; be sure to use it only on raw vegetables.

c. Steam vegetables and eat by mixing in some chopped onion or garlic.

d. Add a little vinegar or some lemon or lime juice and Sprinkle some herbs and spices.

Fruits

Fruits are rich in carbohydrate, vitamins, minerals, and fiber.

Examples of fruits include the following:

- Apples

- Fruit juice

- Strawberries

- Grapefruit

- Bananas

- Raisins

- Oranges

- Watermelon

- Peaches

- Mango

- Guava

What goes into one meal of fruit?

1 small apple or ½ cup juice or 1 grape fruit

1 banana or ½ cup orange juice + ½ cup strawberries

What can you do when trying to have fruits the right way?

a. Eat them without sugar; have them raw if possible.

b. Eat small quantities of fruit.

c. Eating fruit is much better than having fruit juice as fruit has high amounts of fiber in it.

d. Save high-sugar and high-fat fruit desserts only on special occasions.

Milk

Milk is rich in carbohydrate, protein, calcium, vitamins, and minerals.

How do you measure a serving of milk?

1 cup fat free yogurt or 1 cup fat free milk

What are the best and healthiest ways to have milk?

a. Drink fat-free milk

b. Eat low-fat fruit yogurt

c. Use low-fat plain yogurt instead of sour cream.

Meat and Other Items

The meat products you can use and their alternative options include meat, poultry, eggs, cheese, fish, and tofu. Eat them in small amounts every day. These choices have plenty of protein, vitamins, and minerals.

These options include:

- Chicken

- Beef

- Fish

- Canned tuna or other fish

- Eggs

- Tofu

- Cottage cheese

- Cheese

- Pork

- Lamb

- Turkey

How much is in a serving?

a. 1 egg or 2 table spoons of peanut butter

b. 1 slice of turkey + 1 slide of low fat cheese

c. 3 slices of meat, chicken or fish

What are healthy ways to eat them?

a. Buy cuts of beef, pork, lamb that have little fat on them.

b. Eat chicken without the skin.

c. Cook meat in low-fat ways.

d. Add more flavor, use vinegars, lemon juice, ketchup, herbs, and spices.

e. Cook eggs using a non-stick pan.

Fats and Sweets

Take care of the amount of fats and sweets you eat as Fats have lots of calories. Sweets are high in carbohydrates and fat even some contain saturated fats, Trans fats and cholesterol that increase your risk of heart disease. Thus, it will help you to control blood sugar levels.

Some common fats to watch for include:

- Salad dressing

- Oil

- Cream cheese

- Butter

- Mayonnaise

- Avocado

- Olives

Some of the most common types of sweets out there include

- Cake

- Ice cream

- Pie

- Syrup

- Cookies

- Doughnuts

What is a typical serving?

1 cookie or 1 doughnut or 1 tablespoon maple syrup

1 strip of bacon or 1 teaspoon oil

How can I actually eat sweets?

a. Have sugar-free equivalents to whatever you have or use fat free ice cream or frozen yogurt.

b. Don't eat complete desserts; share and eat them with others.

c. Eat small servings of sweets.

   Always talk to your dietician to take care of how much, what and in what quantity you should take sweets.

Diabetes diet - type 2

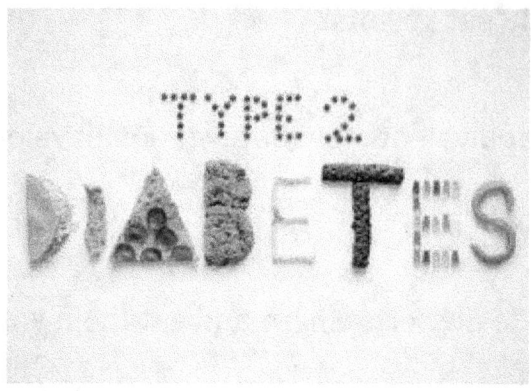

Function

If you have type 2 diabetes, your main focus should be on weight control. Most people who have type 2 diabetes disease are overweight. In fact, this condition is often caused by being overweight.

Improve your blood sugar (glucose) levels by following a meal plan that has:

a. Few calories

b. An even amount of carbohydrates

c. Healthy fats

Foods that are high in monounsaturated fats include peanut butter, almonds, and walnuts. Substitute these foods for carbohydrates but in smaller quantities as they are high in calories.

Improve type 2 diabetes by losing weight and increasing your physical activity levels with activities like engaging in 30 minutes of walking every day.

Children And Type 2 Diabetes

Children with type 2 diabetes have special challenges. Meal plans for children with type 2 diabetes must consider the amount of calories children need to grow.

Kids usually need three smaller meals and snacks to meet their calorie. Most children with type 2 diabetes are obese, thus there is a need to control and manage their weight with increased physical activity.

By making certain Changes in your eating habits along with increases in exercise, a child's blood sugar level will improve. Fewer carbohydrates must also be used with substitutions for potatoes, pasta or rice being used to keep calories and carbs in balance.

Meal Planning

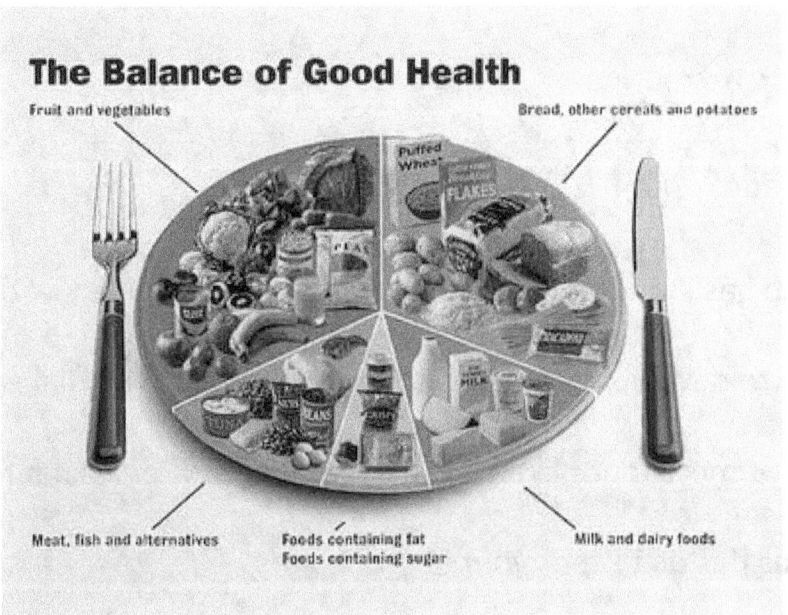

Choose foods with moderate amounts of carbohydrates so that the

blood sugar levels are under good control. To monitor blood sugar

levels regularly is necessary.

Recommendations

Your dietitian can help you to balance the carbohydrates, protein,

and fat in your diet. Do consult him for making your diet plan.

The amount of food you should eat depends on:

a. Your diet

b. Your weight

c. Your exercise routine

d. Your health risks

Everyone has individual needs and likings for food. Work with a dietitian to develop a meal plan for you. A person with diabetes should eat more foods like grains, beans, vegetables than fats and sweets as this diet keeps your heart healthy.

Have the following in your diet:

GRAINS, BEANS, AND STARCHY VEGETABLES

Foods like bread, grains, beans, rice, pasta, and starchy vegetables serve as the foundation of your diet as these are loaded with vitamins, minerals, fiber and carbohydrates.

Eat foods with plenty of fiber. Choose whole-grain foods. bran cereal, brown rice, or beans. Use whole-wheat flours in cooking and baking.

VEGETABLES

Choose fresh vegetables without added sauces, fats, or salt. Opt for more dark green and deep yellow vegetables, like spinach, broccoli, lettuce, carrots, and peppers.

FRUITS

Choose whole fruits than juices as they have more fiber. Citrus fruits, such as oranges, grapefruits are best.

MILK

Choose low-fat milk or yogurt. Yogurt has natural sugar and is low in calories.

MEAT AND FISH

Eat fish and poultry. Bake, roast and broil instead of frying. Remove the skin from chicken and turkey.

FATS, ALCOHOL, AND SWEETS

a. Limit your intake of fatty foods such as hamburgers, cheese, bacon, and butter.

b. If you drink alcohol, limit the amount you have it with a meal.

c. Sweets are high in fat and sugar, so take them in small quantities.

d. Avoid eating too many sweets

e. Split your dessert with others.

f. Eat sugar-free sweets

g. Take the small serving size.

Foods That May Help Control Blood Sugar

Oatmeal

Oatmeal can help control blood sugar as it's high in soluble fiber and is slower to digest and it does not raise your blood sugar as much or as quickly. It's also a steady source of energy that helps to keep you fulfilled for long. Barley is also high in soluble fiber and helps to control blood glucose levels.

Whole grains apart from oat and barley too are good to control the blood sugar levels in your body.

Broccoli, Spinach, and Green Beans

Add no starchy or green leafy vegetables, such as broccoli, spinach, and green beans to your diabetic diet as they are high in fiber and low in carbohydrates, thereby ideal for people with diabetes. Don't cut down on starchy vegetables; include peas, potatoes, corn, winter squash, and lima beans. They give us additional nutrients for maintaining balance in the diet. Vegetables are healthy for people with diabetes as they have more nutrients.

Having vegetables in your diet also helps you to reduce your weight.

Strawberries

Instead of a cookie or candy bar, go for a cup of strawberries but in limited quantities only. They are high in fiber and water and low in calories and carbohydrates.

Salmon and Lean Meats

Meats that are high in protein don't affect blood sugar but must be eaten in proper proportions. Meat is a source of chromium which enables insulin to function properly and also helps to metabolize carbohydrates.

Sparkling Water

Drink sugar-free sparkling water instead of soda. Sparkling water does not contain carbohydrates or calories, thus making it good for maintaining blood sugar levels and managing weight.

Cinnamon

Cinnamon has insulin-like effects that reduce blood sugar levels in people with diabetes.

Low-glycemic diet

A low-glycemic diet is a weight loss diet that controls the body's weight and metabolic process.

The glycemia index (GI) is used to measure short-term changes in blood glucose levels in humans after the intake of carbohydrate-containing foods.

How does carbohydrate counting work?

All food items contain some carbohydrate which increases blood glucose faster than any other food can.

The number of carbohydrates a person can eat each day is determined by:

- Weight and weight loss goals

- How physically active an individual is as physical activity lowers blood glucose levels

- What diabetes medication or insulin they are taking and when

Healthy Diet Basics for Diabetes

A diet for diabetes is a healthy diet that controls calories, fat, sugar, carbohydrates, and salt. The foods that help to control blood sugar are good for everyone. Components of your diet which include the carbohydrate, fat, and protein affect your blood sugar levels.

To make healthy food choices, eat regularly without skipping meals, exercise regularly and take the medicines prescribed by your doctor to keep your blood sugar levels normal.

A proper balanced diet helps people with diabetes to:

a. Control their blood sugar levels

b. Lose weight

c. Control cholesterol levels

d. Reduce the risk of health problems caused by diabetes such as heart disease and high blood pressure

Consult your doctor or dietician who will help you to have a healthy diet plan best suited to your body needs.

General Guidelines for a Diabetes Meal Plan

a. A healthy diet is good for all. The food choices you make must benefit everyone, even if they are not diabetic. Eat plenty of fruits and vegetables that have low fat and sugar.

b. Eat plenty of foods including fruits, vegetables, lean meats, and other forms of protein such as nuts, low-fat dairy products, and whole grains/cereals.

c. Keep your weight in check. Lose weight if you are overweight.

d. Whole grain breads, fruit, and cereal are high in fiber and thus good for you.

e. Eat the same quantity of food every day.

f.   Do not skip meals.

g.   Eat meals and snacks at regular times on all days. If you take a diabetes medicine, eat your meals and take your medicine at the same time every day.

A Diabetes Meal Plan and Sugar

a.   Read food labels. Learn to determine how much sugar or carbohydrates you eat.

b.   Substitute, don't add. Substitute your desert with some other carbohydrate or sugar food.

c.   Sugary foods can be fattening so eat these foods in moderation.

d.   What type of pregnancy diet should I follow if I have gestational diabetes?

e.   If you have gestational diabetes then good nutrition is essential for you. Diabetes is developed when the body cannot produce insulin, which turns sugar into blood glucose.

f. High blood sugar is harmful for the baby and intern for you, so it's essential that you control it.

g. By following a specific meal plan you can control your blood glucose level.

h. Based on your weight, height, physical activity, and the needs of your growing baby make a diet plan with the help of a dietician.

Some general dietary guidelines:

a) Eat a variety of foods that distribute calories and carbohydrates evenly throughout the day. Have balanced meals and snacks.

b) Don't skip meals. To maintain a stable blood sugar level, just be consistent about when you eat meals and the amount of food you eat each day.

c) Eat a good breakfast. Avoid carbohydrates, take proteins and take fruits and juices in small quantities.

d) High-fiber foods such as fresh fruits and vegetables, whole grain breads and cereals should be used in your diet. Keep the sugar level in your body under control and prevent them from going too high.

e) Avoid certain foods all together such as soda, fruit juice, flavored teas and flavored waters, and desserts.

f) Limit the amount of in your diet as it is high in lactose, a simple sugar.

g) Gradually increase your exercising routine in order to maintain the blood glucose levels.

Diet for gestational diabetes

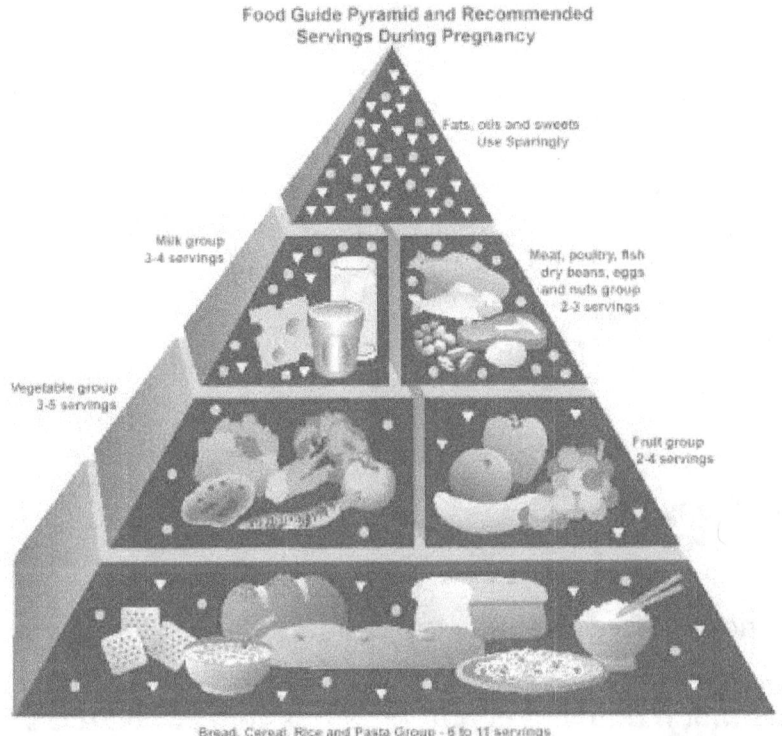

Why do I have to watch what I eat if I have gestational diabetes?

Eating a proper balanced diet is essential during pregnancy and also in order to maintain your blood glucose levels if you have gestational diabetes.

Sugar is the main source of energy for your body. Insulin controls the amount of sugar in your blood in order to turn it into fuel. Hormones during pregnancy reduce the amount of insulin produced, thus the body has to make more of it in order to be able to use it as a fuel.

During gestational diabetes, insulin production is not enough; this can be harmful for the baby. You can control gestational diabetes by using a healthy diet and a regular exercise plan.

How can I change my diet?

If you are not overweight and your blood sugar levels do not show much fluctuation then the condition is not going to be too serious. Still, you will need to watch your diet.

This special diet will guide you which foods you should and shouldn't eat, how much you should be eating and how often you should eat. The diabetic diet is good for everyone for healthy needs.

I've heard about good carbs and bad carbs. What are they?

These are two types of carbohydrates:

a. Complex carbohydrates or starch

b. Simple carbohydrates or sugars

Complex carbohydrates are good carbs, and simple carbohydrates are bad carbs. They include added sugars like honey and natural sugars found in fruits and vegetables.

If you have gestational diabetes and you have drinks and foods that have added sugar then you can experience high fluctuations in your blood glucose levels. Half the energy in our diets comes from carbohydrates. Starchy carbohydrates include:

a. Bread

b. Rice

c. Pasta

d. Grains

e. Potatoes

The wholegrain varieties provide extra fiber important for your digestion.

If you have gestational diabetes then use foods with low numbers of carbohydrates and fats; also, you have to avoid added sugars completely.

What are low GI foods and why are they important?

Low-GI foods are rich in fiber and form an important part of a healthy diet.

Foods with low GI help you to manage gestational diabetes as they take longer for your body to digest and Glucose is released more slowly into the blood.

Foods with a low GI include a few options like these:

a. Pasta made with durum wheat flour

b. Apples, oranges, pears, peaches

c. Beans and lentils

d. Sweet corn

e. Porridge

Consult your doctor or dietitian and get more information on choosing a healthy diet.

How can I improve my diet?

Eat a good breakfast

Eating a good breakfast helps to regulate blood sugar levels in the morning. Have a low-GI breakfast; for instance, having Porridge is a good choice as it releases energy slowly and evenly and maintains your blood sugar levels in range.

Eat a variety of foods during the day

Try to have plenty of foods that are rich in variety so your food is interesting and appealing. Sometimes it helps to use color to help you achieve this by using different foods in different styles and classes.

Eat high-fiber foods

Eat high-fiber foods in plenty as they have a low GI and keeps your blood sugar levels from rising after meals.

High-fiber foods include:

a. Fresh fruit and vegetables

b. Wholegrain breads and cereals

c. Dried peas, beans and pulses

Eat your five a day:

a. Have one fruit with breakfast cereals or porridge.

b. Have a salad in lunchtime with sandwich.

c. Eat vegetables at minimum with your main meal.

d. Eat fruit as snack rather than biscuits or cakes.

Cut down on saturated fats:

a. Use olive oil or sunflower oils for cooking and salad dressings.

b. Have grill foods instead of fried ones.

c. Have nuts and seeds as snacks.

d. Trim fat from meats.

What if I can't control gestational diabetes by diet alone?

Exercise is very important for controlling diabetes as exercise helps to lower blood sugar levels. Any form of exercise like fast walking, swimming, cycling, or even going up and down the stairs are all good ways of exercise as they can increase your heart rate. If diet and exercise are not helping you in a proper way then take the medication with your doctors' prescription or go for an insulin injection.

It's necessary to consult a doctor for help on your diet, exercise or medicines. Your doctor will guide you to inject yourself. That will keep your blood sugar levels in control; you and your baby will be all well.

Dietary Recommendations for Gestational Diabetes

Diabetes that occurs during pregnancy is called gestational diabetes.

Gestational diabetes is diagnosed in about 7 percent of all pregnancies. It develops in the second half of pregnancy and goes away as soon as the baby is born. It is necessary to treat gestational diabetes in order to avoid complications.

For treating gestational diabetes, modify your diet to keep your blood sugar levels in normal range. Women with controlled blood sugar deliver healthy babies without complications.

Try to monitor the amount of carbohydrates in your diet to keep a check on your blood sugar levels. Carbohydrates digest and turn into glucose in the blood and serves as a fuel for your body and nourishment for your baby.

Carbohydrates in Food

Foods with carbohydrates include:

a. Milk and yogurt

b. Fruits and juices

c. Rice, grains, cereals and pasta

d. Breads, tortillas, crackers, bagels and rolls

e. Dried beans, split peas and lentils

Talk with your dietician in order to make a suitable meal plan for yourself according to the carbohydrate requirements for your body. A dietician will also guide you in a plan to count the carbohydrates in your diet.

Limit fruit portions

Fruit is high in natural sugars so stick to a small amount of fruit each day. Avoid canned syrup fruits as they can raise your blood sugar level.

Breakfast matters

Having breakfast is necessary in the morning. Do not skip it. Instead of carbohydrate diet take a meal rich in protein and fiber.

Avoid fruit juice

Fruit has fiber but fruit juice only raises your blood sugar levels so avoid it or else have it diluted with water.

Keep food records

Keep a record of the food you eat and the amount you intake to monitor the carbohydrate in your diet.

Type 2 Diabetes Mellitus Symptoms, Control and Management

What Is It?

Type 2 diabetes is usually caused after middle age but recently with obesity rates increasing it is common to see type 2 diabetes in younger people. Type 2 diabetes is closely related to obesity. Type 2 diabetes is caused when the pancreas fails to produce sufficient amount of insulin in the body to the level of blood glucose in the body.

What happens if insulin does not work effectively?

Insulin's main function is to regulate blood sugar. Once it stops functioning properly, the sugar in the body is not regulated properly and thus, causes an abnormal rise in blood sugar level which leads to diabetes.

Type 2 Diabetes Symptoms

The most common symptoms associated with diabetes are:

a. Excessive thirst

b. Passing of excessive amounts of urine

c. Fatigue

d. Frequent skin infections e.g. boil

e. Itchiness

Diagnosis of Type 2 Diabetes

The doctor first checks for the symptoms and later through a blood sample test the sugar level in the blood from the sample which is taken after an overnight fast.

Preventing Type 2 Diabetes

a. Keep to a healthy weight

b. Eat a healthy diet

c. Ensure adequate levels of daily exercise

How you can help yourself if you have Type 2 diabetes

Help yourself along with your doctor and dietician:

a. If you are overweight, try to lose some weight. Reduction in weight levels helps to reduce the blood sugar levels.

b. Exercise regularly with regard to diabetes as it helps to maintain the blood glucose level in range.

c. Eat healthily: Maintain a healthy diabetic diet.

d. Monitor your blood sugar levels regularly.

Diabetes Treatments: Diet and Exercise

Treatments for Diabetes

- Rapid Acting Insulin
- Short Activity Insulin
- Intermediate Acting Insulin
- Long Acting Insulin
- Ultra Long Acting Insulin
- Insulin Mixtures

- Sulfonylureas
- Meglitinides
- Biguanides
- Thiazolidinediones
- Alpha-Glucosidase Inhibitors

With a proper balanced healthy diet and proper attention to lifestyle can help to prevent type 2 diabetes and keep your blood sugar level in control. Excess weight, hypertension can increase the risk of type 2 diabetes. Lifestyle modification is essential for diabetes type 1 patients too to control their blood glucose levels.

Remember the ground rules

a. Whether you're eating at home or eating out

b. Remember the following

c. Eat a variety of healthy foods.

d. Limit the amount of salt in your diet.

e. Keep portion sizes in check.

Reading food labels: Tips if you have diabetes

Food labels are essential tools for a diabetes meal plan. Try to look for the following when comparing food labels.

a. Start with the list of ingredients in food labels.

b. Keep an eye out for heart-healthy ingredients which include whole-wheat flour, soy and oats. Monounsaturated fats like olive, canola or peanut oils are good for heart health too.

c. Avoid unhealthy ingredients like hydrogenated or partially hydrogenated oil.

d. Ingredients on the product are listed in descending order according to weight. First, the main ingredient is listed followed by other ingredients with decreasing amounts.

e. Look at total carbohydrates, not just sugar. Evaluate the total carbohydrates intake that includes sugar, complex carbohydrate and fiber.

f. Don't miss out on high-fiber foods. High-fiber foods are of great importance in diabetes diet. High fiber foods reduce the absorption of simple carbohydrates.

g. Put sugar-free products in their place. Sugar-free doesn't mean carbohydrate-free. Sugar-free foods play a major role in a diabetes diet. Sugar alcohols contain carbohydrates and calories.

Beware of fat-free products

Fat-free products can still have carbohydrates and calories. You must compare food labels for fat-free and standard products carefully.

Choose healthier fats to lower your cholesterol but watch out as they are often high in calories.

Limit unhealthy fats. Saturated and Trans fats raise the cholesterol level and increase the risk of heart disease.

Questions

I've heard that you shouldn't eat sweet fruits if you have diabetes. Is this true?

It is a myth that some fruits do contain more sugar than others and you should avoid eating them if you have diabetes. The total amount of carbohydrate intake in your body can affect blood sugar levels.

The following fruit servings contain about 15 grams of carbohydrates, a total which is normal for you to indulge in:

1/2 medium banana

1/2 cup (83 grams) cubed mango

1 1/4 cup (190 grams) cubed watermelon

1 1/4 cup (180 grams) whole strawberries

1/3 cup (80 grams) sapodilla (chino)

3/4 cup (124 grams) cubed pineapple

Can I use artificial sweeteners if I have diabetes?

Artificial sweeteners, or sugar substitutes, have less calories and carbohydrates. But still, they must be also used in moderation only.

Is honey a good substitute for sugar?

Both honey and sugar affect your blood glucose levels. Honey has more carbohydrates so even if you plan to substitute sugar and honey there will be no calorie amount that you will be saving. It is necessary for you to maintain your carbohydrate count. So even if you wish to use honey, use it in moderation.

Are late-night snacks a no-no for people who have diabetes?

Late-night snacks add extra calories which lead to weight gain and also to increase your sugar level. You can choose from the following to curb your hunger after meal.

a. A can of diet soda

b. A serving of sugar-free gelatin

c. Five baby carrots

d. Two saltine crackers

e. One vanilla wafer

Diabetes and menopause: A twin challenge

Diabetes and menopause may together cause varied effects on your body. Let's figure out- how to stay in control.

Diabetes and menopause: What to expect

Menopause is the phase when your periods stop.

Changes in blood sugar level

After menopause, hormonal changes trigger fluctuations in the blood sugar level.

Weight gain

Women are likely to gain weight after menopause.

Infections

Before menopause there is risk of vaginal infection due to blood sugar level and after menopause, the risk is much higher.

Sleep problems

After menopause, you experience problems in sleeping that could affect your blood sugar levels.

Diabetes and menopause: What you can do

a. Make healthy lifestyle choices including eating healthy foods and exercising regularly.

b. Measure your blood sugar frequently and ask your doctor about adjusting your diabetes medications.

c. Ask your doctor about cholesterol-lowering medication. Your risk of cardiovascular disease is increased when you have diabetes. Eat healthy foods and exercise regularly to reduce the risk of heart disease which is higher after menopause.

Diabetes and dental care: Guide to a healthy mouth

So, what does brushing and flossing has to do with diabetes?

Let's figure out why dental care is important if you are diabetic and how you should take care of your teeth and gums.

High blood sugar levels can affect your entire body when you have diabetes including your teeth and gums.

It does not matter if you have type 1 diabetes or type 2 diabetes. Control your blood sugar levels because the higher your blood sugar level, the higher your risk of:

Tooth decay (cavities)

When starches and sugars in food and beverages interact with the bacteria in your mouth, plaque forms on your teeth; this can lead to cavities.

Early gum disease (gingivitis)

Diabetes reduces your ability to fight bacteria. It is necessary to remove plaque or it can lead to swollen and bleeding gums.

Advanced gum disease (periodontitis)

Periodontitis is more severe among people with diabetes. It causes you to lose your teeth.

Diabetes and dental care: Guide to a healthy mouth

Make a commitment to managing your diabetes.

a. Monitor your blood sugar level; the better you control your blood sugar level, the less likely you are to have any problems.

b. Brush your teeth at least twice a day. Brush in the morning, at night and after meals and snacks using a soft-bristled toothbrush and fluoride toothpaste.

c. Floss your teeth at least once a day. Flossing removes plaque between your teeth and under your gum line.

d. Schedule regular dental cleanings. Visit your dentist at least twice a year for professional cleanings.

e. Make sure your dentist knows you have diabetes.

f. Look for early signs of gum disease. It is necessary that you report any signs of gum disease like redness, swelling and bleeding gums to your dentist or any other signs and symptoms like a dry mouth, loose teeth or mouth pain.

g. Don't smoke. Smoking increases the risk of diabetes complications including gum disease.

Diabetes and Alcohol

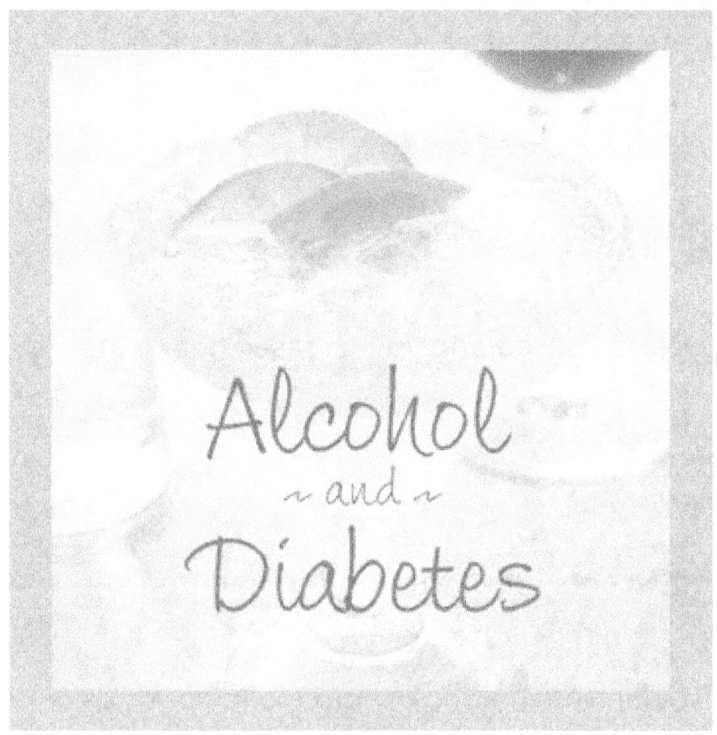

Alcohol contains plenty of calories and can cause your blood sugar levels to rise. If you choose to drink alcohol, only drink it occasionally and when your diabetes and blood sugar levels are well-controlled.

Effects of Alcohol on Diabetes

Moderate amounts of alcohol can cause blood sugar levels to rise; excess alcohol decreases your blood sugar level.

Alcohol stimulates appetite and cause you to overeat and can affect your blood sugar control.

Alcohol affects your judgment and willpower.

Alcohol increases blood pressure.

Alcohol can cause nausea and an increased heart rate.

Diabetes and Alcohol Consumption Dos and Don'ts

People with diabetes who drink should follow these alcohol consumption guidelines:

Do not drink more than two drinks in one day if you are a man or one drink if you are a woman.

Drink alcohol only with meal.

Drink slowly.

Mix liquor with water, club soda, or diet soft drinks.

Food Choices for People with Diabetes

Healthy eating along with regular exercise helps to manage blood glucose levels and reduce your body fats.

What should I eat?

In order to manage your diabetes, your meals should be:

a. An appropriate size.

b. Regular meals intake throughout the day.

c. Low in fat.

d. High fiber carbohydrate foods such as wholegrain breads and cereals, starchy vegetables and fruits.

Fat

Fats have high energy content. Fats taken in moderation and in small amounts add flavor to your food, may improve your health and reduce your risk of heart disease.

Carbohydrate

Carbohydrate foods are the best energy foods. They break down to form glucose. Eating regular meals will help to maintain energy levels without causing any increases in blood glucose levels. If you take diabetes tablets you will require between-meal snacks and all carbohydrate foods are digested to produce glucose. It is best to eat moderate amounts of carbohydrate and include high fiber foods in your diet.

Sugar

Some sugar can be included in your diet plan but it is recommended to avoid high energy foods such as sweets and soft drinks.

Protein

Protein foods provide important nutrients for good health and these do not affect blood glucose levels directly. Protein is found in foods such as lean meat, poultry without the skin, seafood, eggs (not fried),

unsalted nuts and soy products such as tofu.

Alcohol

If you enjoy alcohol, it is generally acceptable to have one standard

drink a day with a meal.

One standard drink can be:

a. 100mL wine

b. 285mL regular beer

c. 30mL spirits

d. 60mL fortified wine

e. 425mL low-alcohol beer (less than 3% alcohol)

Weight management

The first step to cut down your diabetes is to try to manage your

weight.

Try to lose some of it by reducing your calorie intake and following a diet plan with low fat contents. Doing regular exercise such as walking, dancing, riding a bicycle or swimming can help you to lose weight and reduce the risk of diabetes as well.

An example of a meal plan for one day

Make a meal plan and stick to it. The following meal plan can help you to choose what to include:

Breakfast –

3/4 cup of high fiber *breakfast cereal* with *low fat milk*

1 fruit

Tea, coffee or fresh juice

Light meal –

1 sandwich made with 2 slices of *bread*, or 4 dry *biscuits* – preferably *wholegrain* or *whole meal*.

Salad vegetables

A small amount of of lean meat

1 *fruit slice*

Water, tea or coffee

Main meal –

1 *bread roll* or 2 slices of *bread* (preferably *wholegrain* or *whole meal*)

Other vegetables (include freely).

2-4 ounces of lean meat, skinless poultry, seafood, egg, fat reduced cheese

1 piece of *fruit* OR small amount of low fat *yoghurt*

Between-meal snacks

People with diabetes on certain types of tablets need one snack between each meal. It's good if they can include 1 piece of *fruit*, 1 tub of low fat *yoghurt*, 1 cup of low fat *milk,* 1 slice of *wholegrain* bread or 1 slice of *fruit* bread.

www.ingramcontent.com/pod-product-compliance
Lightning Source LLC
Chambersburg PA
CBHW080430290526
45791CB00008BA/2448